Legal & Disclaimer

The information contained in this book is not designed to replace or take the place of any form of medicine or professional medical advice. The information in this book has been provided for educational and entertainment purposes only.

The information contained in this book has been compiled from sources deemed reliable, and it is accurate to the best of the Author's knowledge; however, the Author cannot guarantee its accuracy and validity and cannot be held liable for any errors or omissions. Changes are periodically made to this book. You must consult your doctor or get professional medical advice before using any of the suggested remedies, techniques, or information in this book.

Upon using the information contained in this book, you agree to hold harmless the Author from and against any damages, costs, and expenses, including any legal fees potentially resulting from the application of any of the information provided by this guide. This disclaimer applies to any damages or injury caused by the use and application, whether directly or indirectly, of any advice or information presented, whether for breach of contract, tort, negligence, personal injury, criminal intent, or under any other cause of action.

You agree to accept all risks of using the information presented in this book. You need to consult a professional medical practitioner in order to ensure you are both able and healthy enough to participate in this program.

TABLE OF CONTENTS

INTRODUCTION

Do you feel you could benefit from losing some weight, but for one reason or another you don't get around to it? It could be because of your busy lifestyle, lack of knowledge, plain apathy or an outright dislike or even fear of dieting and exercise. If it has to be done, however, it has to be done.

There is good news and bad news when it comes to weight loss. The bad news is that there is no shortcut. Weight loss, even a small one, requires mental commitment and constant physical follow-up. A mental overhaul and subsequent lifestyle overhaul is required.

Before you run screaming for the door, especially the fridge one, read on for the good news. When I say weight loss requires a mental overhaul, I don't mean you have to change how you think about life just how you think about food and exercise, and even this attitude adjustment is not as drastic as you may fear.

Furthermore, a lifestyle overhaul doesn't mean giving up everything you love and turning into a health freak who nibbles only on carrot sticks and works out all day.

It's all about a mindset adjustment and doing things that are doable, suitable to your lifestyle and smart, and mentally making these small but significant lifestyle changes habits. In this way, while you will have to make some adjustments to your food and eating habits and you won't be able to avoid some form of physical movement, there isn't a huge and daunting 'diet' or 'exercise regimen' to stress about.

A lot of the tricks I will discuss in this book will sound like plain old common sense and are by no means exhaustive. Put together, however, they will instigate a lifestyle avalanche towards good health, which ultimately leads to weight loss.

Take note of the Terrific Tips that I offer for every section. They give you sound-bites of things to do or try to make weight loss fun, easy and sustainable.

CHAPTER 1: INCONVENIENCE YOURSELF

Our everyday activities, done mindfully, burn off significant amounts of calories.

We need to keep burning calories throughout the day. Luckily, everything we do from the moment we wake up to the moment we hit the sack is an opportunity to burn calories. Even if we don't have the time or inclination for a focused 'workout', we're already working out as we go along.

Convenience cancels out exercise opportunities. Make it inconvenient for yourself as much as possible to create mini workouts throughout the day.

Minneapolis fitness trainer Sandra Swami designed a program to encourage busy women to keep active. She suggests you "[stop] using the closest rest room, parking space, or vending machine." Walk to the bathroom at the other end of the building. Get out and physically do your shopping.

Dr. James Levine, M.D., Ph.D of Mayo Clinic has developed a program, NEAT (non-exercise activity thermogenesis), to get people off the couch and into calorie burning mode.

NEAT Tips At Home

• Take the laundry for each person upstairs one at a time.

• Put things away one at a time, instead of gathering everything and distributing them as you go.

• Do as many of your own household chores and repairs as possible.

• Mow your own lawn and wash your own dog and car.

• Hide the remote and physically stand up to change the channel or volume.

NEAT Tips At Work

• Use a small bottle or glass so you have to get up and refill it more often.

• Use a vending machine on another floor.

• Have meetings in the farthest conference room, pace while brainstorming or talking on the phone, throw you rubbish in a general bin, and conduct walk and talk meetings.

NEAT Tips On The Go

• Get off the bus a couple of stops early and walk to your destination.

• Walk instead of using the conveyor belt at airports.

• Go inside the petrol station to pay for you petrol instead of paying at the pump.

NEAT Tips For Running Errands

• Physically go shopping instead of doing online purchasing.

• If you're not buying much, use a shopping basket or bring your own shopping bags to carry around.

• At school pick-up time, get out of the car and walk to the school door.

CHAPTER 2: YOU'VE GOT TO MOVE IT

1. Intensify

Intensify anything you do to turn it into a mini workout. If you're gardening, dig or weed energetically. If you're walking the dog, speed-walk. Even chopping vegetables can be a little workout if you up the energy.

2. Be a Giraffe

By imagining you are a giraffe with a tall straight back, you actually burn calories. According to Taylor-Kevin Isaacs, an exercise physiologist and professor at California State University, Northridge, you should relax your arms by your sides, turning the palms forward. Visualize you are gripping a pen aligned vertically between your shoulder blades. Count to 6, release, then repeat 12 times.

3. (Don't) Sit On It

Swap your chair for a stability ball and gently bounce on it when you are sitting. Cedric X. Bryant, PhD, San Diego's American Council on Exercise's chief exercise physiologist says, "You have to engage the core muscles to maintain stability, so you're getting a great workout right at your desk."

Swami suggests setting a timer to go off hourly. "When it goes off, stand up, and sit down slowly four times," she suggests. "This will boost circulation and give you a nice stretch, and you'll be doing 4 squats an hour, or 32 a day. That's a great way to strengthen your lower body."

4. Take A Walk

Set an alarm to remind you to get up and have a fast-paced walk around the office. You only need five minutes every two hours to make a difference.

Stretch your daily walks to 45 minutes. According to a Duke University study, the normal 30-minute walk will generally prevent weight gain in those who didn't do much other exercise, but a 45-minute walk will actually burn fat. In a study of 10 obese women conducted at the University of Glasgow in Scotland, 20 minutes of walking reduced appetite and increased sensations of fullness as effectively as a light meal.

5. It Ain't Heavy, It's My Bag

Carry your own bags wherever you go. You will strengthen your body and burn calories, according to certified coach Beth Rothenberg, UCLA.

Rothenberg recommends, "[carrying] your groceries, balanced with a bag in each hand, even if you have to make several trips. And pack two smaller suitcases instead of one big one, so you can carry them yourself." Also, try to do some bicep curls while you are carrying your bags.

6. Pump Up The Volume

Dancing is a great workout. Bopping your head, tapping your fingers and toes, shaking your knee to beats that make you happy are feel-good workout sessions that you can do anytime, anywhere. Douglas Brooks, an exercise physiologist and personal trainer in Northern, CA. has a fun way of doing housework: "Turn on some music, add in some vigorous bursts, and enjoy the movement."

7. Every Breath You Take

According to Billy Blanks Jr., creator of the "Dance with Me" classes and DVDs, breathing correctly is a brilliant way to lose weight.

Blanks Jr. says that to benefit your body, you should practice diaphragmatic breathing. Breathe in through your nose, filling your stomach with air. Your stomach should inflate. Release the breath through your mouth, deflating your stomach as the breath is released.

Diaphragmatic breathing burns calories and tones your abdominal muscles through a constant deep core workout. This type of breathing also sends more oxygen to the blood and muscles, replenishing them for a longer workout.

To ensure you're breathing correctly, lie on your back. Put your hand on your stomach and breathe, raising your hand up. Open your mouth a little and exhale slowly, feeling your stomach flatten again. Repeat the process 35 times.

8. Laugh It Off

Did you know that a good belly chuckle is a great abdominal workout? It is the perfect cardiovascular workout that raises the heart rate and pumps circulation up.

Stafford University's Dr. William Fry states, "Laughing heartily five times a day has the same beneficial effects as ten minutes on a rowing machine."

9. Step Up

We see steps everywhere … use them! It's an instant cardio, leg and buttock workout. Go up and down some stairs for 10 minutes every day. That's all The Centre for Disease Control says your body needs to lose weight if your eating habits stay the same.

CHAPTER 3: LESS IS MORE

Keeping your workout the right length is key for fat burning. Health, fitness, safety and wellness consultant Dr. Marc Tinsley warns that exercise in excess of 45 minutes can actually trigger cortisol production, which in turn triggers fat production.

Split a 60-minute workout into two 30-minute sessions with a short break in between, Tinsley suggests. Then your body will work as a "fat-burning machine," Tinsley said.

Metabolic training works well, in light of this. Combining cardio, power, endurance, mobility and whole body strength into one 30-minute workout, it continues to burn calories even after the workout is over. It also builds muscle and jumpstarts the metabolism.

Below, I've given you a sampling of the exercises. For the full workout, go to http://www.livestrong.com/slideshow/557797-the-16-most-effective-fat-loss-moves-no-equipment-required/#slide=1.

Metabolic Training

Perform these exercises for 30 seconds at a time initially. Gradually add 5 to 10 seconds as your metabolic conditioning improves, peaking at 60 seconds. To burn the most fat, keep your heart rate cranked up, and torch the most calories, only rest for 30 seconds or less between movements. Finally, alternate between working your upper body and lower body, or your front and back.

1. Ground Zero Jump

Place your feet hip-width apart. Point your toes forward and flex your unlocked knees. With a flat back, push your buttocks back to jut out and extend your arms pointing backward like a skier going downhill. Squat down slowly, then push your hips forward with high energy, so you end up standing straight. At the same time, swing your arms forward to chest level. Repeat.

Starting off: - Go slowly.

Getting better: - Speed up. End up with arms extended over your head, standing on your toes.

Ultimate workout: - Lift off your feet a little with the upward movement.

This is a lower-impact jumping activity that exercises your whole body, focusing on your backside, hips and core muscles. It burns calories but is gentle on the joints. Targeting fast-twitch muscle fibers, ground zero jumps work the best to improve your athleticism, metabolism and heart rate.

2. Predator Jacks

Keep your feet together and place your palms together in front of you with straightened but unlocked arms. Jump and part your feet, then bend the knees and lower into a squat. At the same time, pull your arms apart, pulling your shoulder blades back until your arms line up with your shoulders. Lean over a little to one side, then the other, then back to center and stand up to your beginning position.

Speed up and intensify as you go.

This exercise, reminiscent of how the predators in the movie "Predator" moved, is a great metabolic mobilizer. In just a minute, it energizes the nerves between your mind and muscles and loosens up the normally knotted up areas in the ankles, hips and upper back.

3. Skater Jumps

Put your weight onto one leg and bend that knee slightly. Bend your other knee slightly too, so that foot hovers above the ground. Jump off the grounded foot and land softly on the other. Count to one with your hips back and low, then jump back on the other foot.

Intensify the workout by pretending you are a giant stuck in a house and keep your head and hips down.

A great workout to exercise your legs and lungs in a rush while still being gentle to your heart. Replicating the movements of speed skating, this move touches the rarely exercised areas of your hips that deal with side-to-side motion.

4. Blast-Off Push-Ups

Align your hands directly beneath your shoulder as if you're going to do push-ups. Tighten your abs and glutes and make sure there's a straight line from head to heels. Slowly push the hips back, keeping your lower back flat so your legs bend about 90 degrees and your head comes behind your hands. Count to one, then in an explosive action straighten your knees, ankles and hips into a straight line and pull with your lower back, so you end up in the resting position of a push-up. Tuck your elbows in as you go down.

Starting off: - Don't do a pushup.

Ultimate workout: - Move your feet closer together and do the push-up.

This movement burns fat off every part of the body. You practice moving explosively at your hips while keeping your lower back steady which results in great core stability, and the pushing and pulling at the upper body firms the shoulders. The heart rate is also pumped up.

CHAPTER 4: BE A COUCH POTATO

It's possible to lose weight as you watch TV! Use those pesky 3-minute commercial breaks to get active. With six commercials, you get nearly half an hour of activity while you're waiting for your show.

Prevention's fitness advisor Wayne L. Westcott, PhD, of Quincy, MA. says that the couch potato workout is suitable for anybody of any fitness level. It adds on to overall daily activity, so helps to keep the metabolism working. As with all exercise, put as much intensity as you can into them.

First Break – Couch Pushup

Chest, back of the arms.

Face the couch and kneel 2 feet away from it. Cross your ankles and lean your hands on the couch, shoulder-width apart. Bend your arms until your chest touches the couch, count to ten, and push up again. Do all movements slowly and deliberately.

Do 10 to 15 reps. Round off with some jumping jacks.

Second Break – Side Crunches

Obliques.

Lie on your side and place your legs together, bending the knees a little. Bend the topmost arm to point the elbow to the ceiling, placing that hand behind your head. Wrap the bottom-most arm around your waist. Squeeze the oblique muscles on your topmost side to bring that shoulder up to touch your rib cage to your hip. Count to ten then slowly release.

Do 10 to 15 reps. Switch sides. Do some crossover punches by standing and punching the air with alternate fists, twisting from your waist to reach your fist across your body.

Third Break – Armchair Stands

Front of the thighs, buttocks.

Sitting on the edge of the couch, open your legs to shoulder-width. Push your feet into the floor. Stand up slowly, keeping your arms by your sides. Tighten you buttock muscles on the way up. Keep your back straight and you abdominals tight. Count to ten and slowly go down again. Just before your buttocks touch the chair, lift up again.

Do 10 to 15 reps. Walk briskly around the room or up and down the stairs.

Fourth Break – Armchair Dips

Back of the arms.

Sit on the edge of the couch and spread your arms out on the couch on either side of you. Put your feet together, pointing forwards. Step forward until your buttocks are off the couch, and your knees are bent at 90-degrees. Bend your elbows to point backward and lower yourself until you feel the stretch. Count to ten and slowly raise yourself up.

Do 10 to 15 reps. Circle your fists in front of you as if you are boxing a punching bag.

Fifth Break – Leg-up Couch Crunches

Abdominals.

Lie on your back, bend your knees and lift your feet up, so your legs form a right angle. Place your hands behind your head and push your lower back into the couch. Slowly pull your whole upper body up towards your knees, count to ten and slowly go down again.

Do 10 to 15 reps, and then stand up and lift one leg up, knee bent. Touch that knee with the opposite bent elbow and switch.

Sixth Break – Scissors

Inner and outer thighs.

Lie on your back and place your hands palm down under your buttocks. Lift your legs to point to the ceiling and bend your knees slightly, flexing your feet. Slowly push your legs sideways away from each other until you feel a stretch. Count to ten, and slowly close your legs.

Do 10 to 15 reps. Stand up and do side slides. Place one foot out to the side and slide the other foot over to place next to it. Swap feet.

CHAPTER 5: YOU ARE WHAT YOU EAT

Just as movement is essential for weight loss, eating right is too, as what we put into our body directly affects our weight. I am not going to advocate calorie-counting because, important as it is, good calorie intake can be achieved by just tweaking your diet. It's about small tweaks in our lifestyles, not scary lists of dos and don'ts.

1. Keep It Natural

It's obvious to keep it natural when selecting foods that will aid in weight loss. The closer it is to how nature intended, the less has been added. It is also more nutritious, therefore probably more satisfying. Opt for fruits, raisins, nuts, vegetable sticks rather than cookies or even granola bars.

2. Pump Up The Fiber

Both soluble and insoluble fiber aid in weight loss. Soluble fiber soaks in water and forms a gel which slows digestion down, satiating you faster and keeping you satiated for longer.

Insoluble fiber serves as a laxative by adding bulk to your stool, clearing your digestive system and preventing bloating. Both forms of fiber regulate sugar absorption into the bloodstream, staving off obesity and diabetes.

Fiber is what plants are made of, so most natural, unprocessed foods have it, like vegetables, whole grains, vegetables, beans, and fruits. The American Dietetic Association recommends at least five servings of vegetables a day.

3. Make Like A Cow

A salad a day keeps the pounds away. It fills you up with vitamins, minerals, and dietary fiber and stops the stomach from growling for less beneficial food.

Make healthy salads with flavorsome yet guilt-free ingredients like rocket leaves, nuts and fruits. Make your own dressings too.

4. Don't Only Make Like A Cow

Although salads are great, it's a bad idea to only eat salad at mealtimes, says Manuel Villacorta, a dietician and American Dietetic Association spokesperson. Salad does not do enough to lower levels of ghrelin, the hunger hormone. "If you're not eating enough, you're not lowering your ghrelin amounts, and you'll eat more later," he said.

Villacorta says you need healthy carbohydrates to fill you up. He recommends pairing salad with a healthy sandwich or some nutritious soup. You can also add fruits, grains, pasta or bread to your salad.

5. White Fright

We all know simple carbohydrates like those in white flour and white sugar causes chaos to our blood sugar and weight. Since you need carbohydrates to bulk up your meals, replace them with harder to metabolism complex carbohydrates like brown rice and whole-grain bread.

Add less starchy carbohydrates to your meal and bulk it up with vegetables. Carrots, broccoli, cauliflower, tomato or even mushrooms to fill up your plate and stomach.

6. Variety Is The Spice Of Life

Spices like cloves and pepper give your palate a zing and can help you shed pounds by curbing your appetite. These findings were based on research by The Endocrine Society that showed the weight loss of a group of people who added calorie- and salt-free flavorings to their food. Spicy foods also fire up your digestive juices to burn more calories.

Stronger flavored foods also have a psychological effect that's great for weight loss. According to Alan Hirsch, M.D., founder of Chicago's Smell & Taste Treatment and Research Foundation, "The flavors made people focus on the sensory characteristics of the food - its smell and taste." Basically, when food is tastier, you tend to enjoy it more and feel full faster.

7. Say No To Numbers

Pay attention to the ingredient list of packaged foods. Avoid foods whose ingredients have numbers in their names. These are full of fat and preservatives, according to Dr. Carson Liu, a Los Angeles bariatric surgeon.

"If you're trying to lose weight, it's very, very difficult to do so with processed foods because they have so many carbs, sugars, and hidden ingredients, " Liu said.

8. Nix The Corn Syrup

Scientific research by a group from Princeton University shows that a beverage sweetened with high-fructose corn syrup (HFCS) will push your weight up, as opposed to a beverage sweetened with the same amount of sugar.

This can be explained by the molecular makeup of the 2 sweeteners. While both are made up of fructose and glucose, the two compounds are bound up tighter in sugar, so they need more energy to break down. In corn syrup, they are separate so don't require as much energy to metabolize. Check your food's ingredients and avoid those with corn syrup.

9. Junk The Junk

We all know junk food is bad for us, but an alarming new study laid out in March 2010's Nature Neuroscience journal indicates the possibility that junk food can be addictive, affecting the brain in a similar way to drug abuse.

In the study, rats were offered as much junk food as they wanted. An obvious result was that the animals became obese, but a disturbing side effect was that two drug addiction indicators also appeared.

Dopamine receptors, which are crucial to the brain's reward system, vanished which meant the body now needed more food to feel full. The subject's behavior was also altered, and they craved they foods, not even stopping when they were warned of punishment. This reflects how compulsive eaters and addicts behave, according to study researcher Paul Kenny of Scripps Research Institute in Florida.

10. Berry Good

If you are craving for something sweet, consider berries – especially lingonberries. Scandanavian lingonberries are similar to cranberries but are packed with more nutrition.

In a study conducted by the Journal of Nutrition and Metabolism, lingonberries nearly negated the effects of a high-fat diet. It stopped weight gain and kept blood sugar levels even. This study was conducted on mice, however, so further study is required on humans.

One definite benefit of lingonberries is that they contain high levels of the polyphenol antioxidant.

11. Release The Fat

If you must indulge, opt for fat-releasing foods. Certain foods may seem high in calories, but they have inbuilt fat releasers.

Eggs have fat releasing protein while part-skim ricotta cheese has fat releasing calcium. Dark chocolate is slightly higher in calories but is packed with fat releasers.

Additionally, a study from the University of Tennessee showed that those who were already losing weight and took yoghurt three times a day lost even more body fat.

Researchers also found that low-fat dairy foods contain a type of calcium that sparks off hormones that inhibit the production of fat cells. It also boosts fat breakdown.

12. Water Explosion

Go for foods that are water-rich. Research from Pennsylvania State University shows foods like tomatoes, cucumbers and zucchinis will fill you up so that you don't consume other higher - calorie foods.

Terrific Tips

Breakfast

• Have steel-cut or rolled oats, or whole-grain cereal 5 times a week.

• Sprinkle on frozen lingonberries.

Lunch

• Filling vegetables include potatoes, sweet potatoes, carrots, broccoli, and tomatoes.

• Look for low-fat salad dressings.

• Strongly flavored cheese like sharp cheddar is lower in fat.

• Go for extra-lean (85% lean) ground beef.

• Spice up with onions, garlic, hot peppers, horseradish or other strong spices.

Snacks

• Go for grapefruit, oranges, cantaloupe, apricots, peaches and berries.

• Applesauce is a naturally sweet substitute for fats. Use it to replace half the amount of fat required when baking.

• Mix fresh nuts with raisins, seeds, and dried fruits.

• Choose frozen yoghurt over ice-cream.

Dinner

• Pre-prepare salad makings, frozen vegetables, chicken breasts and even frozen pizza dough for a quick, nutritious dinner.

• Stock some healthy low-fat frozen dinners for emergencies.

CHAPTER 6: YOU ARE HOW YOU EAT

1. Put On That Apron

Do it right, do it yourself. You will then be in complete control of what goes into your mouth. Food made outside is loaded with oil, fats, salt, and preservatives. Portions are also often too large.

Browse recipe books or websites to find easy appetizing and nutritious recipes. Plan your weekly meals so you can shop for everything you need in one go. It's a lot easier to be motivated if you aren't bogged down at the wrong time.

2. Take It Slow

It's well-known that you will lose weight if you eat slowly. This is because the brain needs 20 minutes to get the "full" message from the stomach. Slowing your fork down will give the brain the catch-up time it needs.

Consciously prolong time between bites. Put your fork down while you are chewing, and count your chews. An additional benefit is that your food is more thoroughly digested.

3. One Step At A Time

Drastic food intake cuts will probably backfire in the long run because you might mentally resist it. Cut down in increments. Have one less snack or one less manufactured beverage a day. You will find that your body and mind will not even miss it, eventually.

4. Be Mindful

When you eat mindlessly, the food becomes empty calories. It's tempting to watch television or otherwise occupy yourself during mealtimes, but Marissa Lippert, a New York City registered dietician and nutrition counselor, advises you to put everything aside and really focus on what's on your plate.

By acknowledging and appreciating the taste, color, texture and presentation of your food, you will be more deeply satisfied and psychologically satiated faster.

5. Change It Up

New research out of Cornell University advocates altering your meals' surroundings. Eat your lunch elsewhere in the office, or even outside.

At home, make up a plate to take to the table, forcing you to get up and walk to the kitchen for seconds. This often makes people think twice about another round. At the very least, your body has time to signal that it's full to the brain.

6. Re-lay The Table

Table setting can affect how much you eat. Use smaller dinner plates and your plate will seem more full. Even downsize your cups and glasses for anything other than water.

Color affects our moods and the way we perceive things. Choose a dish that is a different color to your food. Studies show that we tend to eat more when the food and the plate are the same color. The color blue has been known to suppress the appetite, so try to lay your table with something blue.

7. Just Do It

Counter-intuitive to those who are trying to lose weight, one piece of advice has been to just give in to your cravings, within reason. The more you resist the urge, the more it will psychologically eat at you (pun intended).

To counter the damaging effects of craving fulfillment, make smart choices - dark chocolate instead of a hot fudge sundae, for example.

8. Sniff It

This piece of advice might seem weird, but when you feel hungry, grab an apple, a banana or a peppermint and sniff it. An experiment conducted by Alan R. Hirsch, M.D., neurological director of Chicago's Smell & Taste Treatment and Research Foundation on 3,000 volunteers showed that if they sniffed something healthy when they were hungry, the olfactory satisfaction was enough to signal to the brain that they were full. The result was that they ate less.

More Terrific Tips

• Fix lunch the night before and brown bag it.

• Keep gravies, sauces and dips on the side so you can dip your fork into them before spearing your food.

• When you're done with dinner, clean up, take what you need (like water), and close the kitchen for the night.

• If you face a mirror while you eat, you tend to eat less. Your reflection reminds you of your weight loss goals.

• Use your non-dominant hand to eat. You will take more time to scoop your food, and you will be forced to be mindful of every mouthful you take.

• Order small. Studies show that we normally only eat what's in front of us because by the time we order or get up for seconds, our brains will have received the "full" signal.

CHAPTER 7: THE RIGHT TIME

Some medical experts have examined weight loss by eating specific foods at specific times of the day. If you eat certain foods at certain times, you maintain your blood sugar levels, which helps your body to feel fuller.

RealAge's article "Six Meal Diversity Deal", recommends six smaller meals of highly nutritious, filling food consisting of unsaturated fats, high fibre, and high protein. This will keep your energy levels high and your insulin and blood sugar levels balanced.

1. No Skipping

A good breakfast triggers the metabolism early in the day so that the body will burn calories more efficiently. It also sets the scene for healthier eating habits and food choices.

If you skip breakfast, you are hungry by lunchtime, which leads to overeating. It also promotes snacking to stave off the hunger pangs, and usually by these times we crave for carbohydrate heavy foods. Squeeze in a simple, quick, but nutritious breakfast sometime early in the morning.

2. Pump Up The Protein

Protein is the most filling food source, alongside fat. Good solid doses of natural protein actually promote weight loss as you feel satiated for longer.

Eat a good breakfast that includes natural protein, then opt for lighter meal choices the rest of the day. Maria Fernandez, senior researcher at the University of Connecticut, said to LiveScience, "[this] is especially good when people are trying to lose weight. If you eat a high-protein meal at breakfast, it helps decrease your appetite for the rest of the day.

3. Don't Wait Too Long

Lippert points out a mistake that many dieters make - waiting too long between mealtimes, which makes them crave energy-rich carbs. They choose foods that fill up the body quickly, not thinking about healthy options or portions. The body's metabolism might also be affected.

Space your meals and snacks out to be 3 hours apart, Lippert recommends. Your body will get used to a predictable routine and won't have energy cravings. You will also be able to "tap into your hunger and satiety cues", according to Lippert, and match your intake to your needs.

When you have fixed mealtimes, your body's ghrelin (hunger hormone signaler) spikes at expected mealtimes, so if you eat early, you might still feel hungry. Have healthy snacks available to stem being moody.

Terrific Tips

Breakfast

- 1 cup unsweetened oats (fiber)

- Fresh or dried fruit (fiber, vitamins)

- 1 glass skim milk (fat-releasing calcium)

- 1 bowl multi-grain cereal

- Fresh or dried fruit (fiber, vitamins)

- 1 bowl low-fat yoghurt (fat-releasing calcium, good fat)

- 1 handful unsalted nuts (energy)

- Non-sweetened instant oatmeal (fiber)

Lunch

- An apple before your meal (fiber, filling)

- Avocado for a lunch on the go (good fats, filling)

- Almond butter (stabilizes blood sugar)

- Whole wheat bread (fiber)

Snacks

- Watermelon / cantaloupe / watery fruit (hydrating diuretic, filling)

- 1 hour before working out - Greek yoghurt (fat-releasing calcium, good fat)

- Frozen berries (energy)

Late Night Snack

- Carrot or celery sticks (alkaline, easily digestible)

Dinner

- Early, small and nutritious meals (digestion time before bed)

CHAPTER 8: DRINK IT OFF

The scary thing is that you can actually consume more calories in a day from beverages than from food. Go natural - which is true for anything you consume. The more manufactured ingredients are in something, the less it is good for you and can drive your weight up.

1. H2O

Water doesn't melt fat, but it has zero calories and benefits the body in so many ways.

More interestingly, did you know that sometimes when you feel hungry it's actually because your body needs water, not food. We often confuse thirst signals for hunger ones and mistakenly eat.

Another reason that water is a weight loss elixir – it keeps our bodies properly hydrated for optimum processing. In digestion, this means food is moved through the system more promptly, avoiding bloating.

Do take note, however, that water is not filling enough to substitute a meal. Hunger and thirst are processed differently, and water won't do the trick of keeping you full.

2. Fight The Fizz and Tizz

As with processed foods, manufactured beverages contain empty calories and excess sugar. Even so-called 'healthy' fruit juices should be taken in moderation and only freshly squeezed or juiced.

The same goes for coffee - avoid those popular specialty blends and stick to fresh-brewed. If you must have soda, opt for the diet varieties. Beware of diet options of anything. However, the sweeteners used to flavor them actually have high glycemic content. There is even controversy over 'natural' sweeteners like stevia.

Alcohol does even more damage weight-wise. It has a high-calorie count and slows the metabolism down.

3. Salt Water Wells In My Cup

Salt has been vilified in health circles, but it does have its benefits, especially when it's added to water.

"Water needs electrolytes like sodium, potassium, and chloride to be best absorbed," Jenny Westerkamp, an R.D. in Chicago, says. Westerkamp suggests pinching a little pure Celtic sea salt or real salt into your water bottle or glass. "The electrolytes in the salt will push water into the cells where they need to be, rather than letting the water get flushed out, causing you to go to the bathroom every other minute."

Two other benefits of drinking salty water? An energy spike and a full stomach, therefore less chance of snacking.

4. Matcha, Matcha, Matcha

Matcha is a powdered Japanese green tea. We all know the benefits of green tea, one of which is the high levels of epigallocatechin Galgate (EGCG), which retards fat cell growth.

5. Milk It

A study done be researchers at the Nutrition Institute of the University of Tennessee showed that 3 servings of dairy added to a reduced-calorie diet aided weight loss.

One reason for this might be because calcium is stored in fat cells and the more calcium in the cells, the more of its fat will be released.

Additionally, calcium binds to fat in the GI tract, blocking its absorption.

Terrific Tips

• When you feel hungry, sip some water first.

• Choose locally produced organic milk - non-organic milk contains fattening hormones.

• Grass-fed cows milk contains more conjugated linoleic acid (CLA) which burns fat quicker.

• Skim milk has 0 grams of fat, but the same levels of calcium and vitamin D. If it's too watery, try two percent or non-fat powdered milk.

• Try evaporated skim milk as an alternative to cream.

CHAPTER 9: KITCHEN OVERHAUL

Obviously what you do in the kitchen also makes a difference to your weight. Fry, grill or bake? What dry ingredients do you stock in the pantry?

1. Location, Location, Location

Consider rearranging your whole kitchen to make things less convenient for yourself. If you can, set up your workstation further away from your stove and fridge or rearrange things, so you have to move around the kitchen to get things done.

2. Ditch The Machines

Do all your cooking manually to expend more energy. When you bake, use a spatula to stir. Wash your dishes by hand. Intensify your actions, tense your muscles and turn on the music to bop along as you cook. The added benefit of dancing is that your meals pick up positive vibes.

3. Kitchen Weights

Buy heavy, good-quality utensils so it takes more energy to lift and use them. Lift your pots and pans as often as possible, and throw in some squats while you're at it.

4. The (Wo)man With The Plan

Make a meal plan at the end of every week for the upcoming week. When you're satisfied with your plan, draw up a shopping list of all the items you need to ensure you have everything at hand for a week's worth of healthy eating.

5. The Need For Speed

If you really are pressed for time, go for frozen vegetables and fruits. This way, you won't be demoralized about preparing your own meals. Save chopping and bopping for the weekends.

Another great reason to go for frozen produce is that it may be more nutritious since it is picked and frozen at the optimal time.

More Terrific Tips

• Place the kitchen bin as far away from your workstation as possible.

• Change your bin to an old-fashioned one that you have to physically lift the lid off.

• Practice using your foot to hook the lid handle to lift it.

• Rearrange your shelves so that the often-used items are on the top shelves.

• Store prepared meals in single-serve containers.

CHAPTER 10: THE ALTERNATIVE

Although this book deals primarily with foods and exercises, this last chapter will look at some alternative weight loss methods. As always, consult a reliable expert before you start anything.

1. Stick A Needle In It

Acupuncture is an ancient Chinese healing method that balances the functions of the organs by using needles to stimulate the body's energy points.

Douglas Eisenstark L.Ac, an acupuncturist who has served as Clinic Supervisor at Emperor's College and Yo-San University, says, "Weight loss is a part of the 'middle burner' or the spleen, stomach and liver organ systems of Chinese Medicine." When those meridians are simulated, digestion is promoted, and excess is cleared from the system. Stress, which is also addressed by the same meridians and is a large cause of over-indulgence, is also balanced.

2. Can I Get A Remedy

Chinese medicinal herbs go hand in hand with acupuncture to balance the body's energy. Traditional Chinese Medicine practitioners consult with and prescribe for each person differently, according to their specific body energy makeup and dis-balances. Everyone's trigger for weight gain is different, and so is treated accordingly.

3. Aromatherapy

The use of aromatherapy oils may or may not directly cause weight loss, but it does affect our state of mind, which weight gain is very much tied up to. As the body needs to be balanced, so does the mind, and that's where aromatherapy can help. One can deal with mental imbalances that lead to overeating by balancing them with specific blends of oils. A blend of rose, sandalwood, and orange can help alleviate anxiety and depression, for example. A blend that addresses loneliness is rose, frankincense and bergamot.

4. Supplements

Bear in mind that many supplements purported to promote weight loss have yet to be studied thoroughly. Having said that, some supplements to take note of are:

1. 7-Keto-DHEA

This chemical occurs naturally in our body, derived from DHEA hormone metabolism. It boosts weight loss by speeding the metabolism up.

7-Keto-DETA, taken together with exercise and a well-controlled diet has shown to promote weight loss. However, The Natural Medicines Comprehensive Database says the evidence is not enough to be conclusive either way. It seems to be safe - no significant side effects were observed after taking it for 28 days.

2. Vitamin D

Studies have shown that vitamin D controls "insulin sensitivity", how well body cells respond to insulin. If the cells are more sensitive, the body will absorb and burn more calories. If they are less sensitive, it will store more calories in its fat cells.

Parathyroid hormone (PTH) levels rise when vitamin D is low, causing a domino effect. Sugar is then converted into fat and stored, according to Michael B. Zemel, PhD, Nutrition Institute director at the University of Tennessee in Knoxville.

Vitamin D deficiency might also cause production of less leptin, which tells the brain to stop eating, to be secreted.

3. Alli (Non-Prescription Orlistat)

It has been claimed that Alli decreases dietary fat absorption, but more study needs to be done into its specific benefits. It has been observed to have a moderate effect on weight loss but does not seem as effective as Xenical, the prescriptions-strength version.

Some side effects observed have been loose oily stool, difficult-to-control bowel movements and very rare but reported cases of serious liver damage.

CONCLUSION

Now that you've seen how easy it can be to lose weight, I hope you take it to heart and start trying at least some of these techniques.

I have tried to present no-fuss, no-equipment workouts that you can do anytime, anywhere, and I hope that you will come to think of them as fun (you must admit, bopping around with the vacuum, pretending you are Beyonce IS fun!)

It really isn't hard to be NEAT, although you might have to get used to deliberately inconveniencing yourself. You might find rearranging your environment initially troublesome, but once it's done, you will quickly slip into the easy new habits and slip off the pounds.

As to tweaking your diet, that's exactly what it is … tweaking your favorite meals by swapping some of the ingredients with healthier options. I've even given you some tips on how and when to eat to maximize weight loss. All you need to do it take some of the suggestions on board and, again, make them into habits.

As I mentioned before, I've only presented a small range of suggestions to lose weight with minimal exercise and diet tweaking. There are a whole plethora of other methods out there, just remember that, whatever you decide to take on board, think about whether it makes sense, is doable for you, sustainable and vetted by an expert.

I wish you all the best in your quest for a healthy, happy, wholesome body!